Healthy Cooking, Healthy Living on $176 a month: my story

By

Susan Devine Napoli

"Where there is a will, there is a way."

This book is based on information I was given by my medical doctor and is an account of my progress through the confusing literature on nutrition and fitness. I do not take responsibility for anyone's progress but mine. This is a program I devised for myself and share it in effort to say it is possible to become healthy and fit on a low budget using simple resources. If you choose to use any of the information in this book the responsibility is entirely yours. Your results may vary.

Contents

◊◊◊

Introduction

$176 a month is not much money for healthy food for one person. It is easy to spend quite a lot on food. There are so many choices for those who seemingly have the money and those who do not seem to not have that choice. It is not true. I found the nutritional "gold" for myself in discount foods and simple exercise.

Years ago, I heard this: "The answer to the problem is not more money." I don't know where I got that but I know it to be true. When I accept powerlessness I get nothing. America was built on ingenuity, with empty wallets and full hearts. Eighty-one companies started their businesses during the Great Depression that still exist today, examples of overcoming in times of adversity. There are many such examples in America.

I decided to tap into the ingenuity and thrive. I am healthier than I ever thought possible. I reduced my risk of heart disease, high blood pressure, and type 2 diabetes by cooking for myself healthy meals and doing daily simple exercise that I love.

I found the answer for myself and decided to share it. I used my own ingenuity to solve the problem by collecting and going through information and tease out the answer for myself. I spent quite a lot of time working on it, and I wrote this book. Information + time + Amazon print on demand, has made it possible for me to get this to you without a big bill for me. It's beautiful how ingenious this is. More money was not the answer to my problem.

My hope is that you might find a few pieces to your own puzzle in these pages. It is a program I developed for myself. No program is perfect for everyone. I decided to tailor the information I found to suit my own health needs together with information from my doctor. She supplies the data on my general health. I do the work of taking good care of myself.

This is what I needed for this process:

A pair of walking shoes: nothing fancy, something that has support for my feet.

A library card: this gives me access to a computer, cookbooks, and online help on you tube.

Time and supplies to do the things I loved to do. Namely, painting, sewing, and writing. Going places around town like parks, thrift shops, and antique stores.

Willingness to make a few changes: surprisingly, this was the hardest part.

A Sidekick glucose monitoring system with separate sharps and pen, the cheapest on the market to date. (available at Walmart)

Let me tell you the story of how I did it for myself in weeding through the incredible amount of information, misinformation and hype. It was so confusing. I got lost in the weight loss industry and found my way out. I spent too much money, time, and energy for what I could have for free.

Susan

My Story

How I found the Information

"I can't afford to eat healthy," was the complaint again and again in my college class on Wellness of the Young Child at the community college I worked at preparing teachers. The point of the class was to learn to create a healthy environment for children in the child care and school settings. I was only required to have taught children and have a Master's degree in Early Childhood Education to teach the class. As I taught the class, I found myself in over my head with trying to teach this class. It became evident over time that I could not really separate the care of the children and the health of the adult caring for them. In order for the adults to monitor the children in their care well, they had to come face to face with their own wellness or lack thereof. It made me have to come face to face to mine too and being 70 pounds overweight at my heaviest.

"Of course you can eat healthy," I replied.

"How?" was the question that was a challenge and a question I was searching for too. I had only part of the answer and I gave that to them. It wasn't enough. I knew it. They knew it. They had tried like me and were searching.

We cooked fresh vegetables I bought at Walmart when I figured out vegetables were a key part of healthy living, lots of them. Some tried something new. Some didn't. I discovered how very personal food choices were. It's no wonder what I tried didn't work for me and for them either. Everyone was searching. I brought in speakers that gave us the same information as in the textbook and answered the hard questions.

I have been working on it lately for me. The course does not exist anymore but the question still remained even though I don't even work there anymore. Good questions are like that. I have come up with an answer that I am satisfied with, finally. I got a handle on my own wellness.

I had to comb through all the fads and sensational information to find out how to eat really heathy on an extremely tight budget. There is a lot of really bad information out there and recipes that didn't work for me. I got fooled a lot.

I am not a nutritionist. Just a teacher, mom, new grandmother, and a retired early childhood professional with a master's degree who wanted to get healthy. I used the skills I learned about doing research to find my answer. It was a field I was unfamiliar. That made it difficult. I had tried several programs preceding finding the answer for myself: Richard Simmons food mover, Bob Green, Weight Watchers and a few more. I was successful every time. I even achieved a lifetime membership at Weight Watchers by losing 56 pounds. It did not make me healthier, according to my doctor's reports. I couldn't understand why. Each program gave me more to the puzzle I was to solve. I couldn't stick with these programs long term.

I was frustrated by buying books that looked good but had too many ingredients, too complicated a process for me as a working mom at the end of the day. When I was not working, I didn't want to spend the whole day cooking just to be healthy. I found there were ingredients I didn't know what they were but recommended. I went to the store and found I could not afford them.

I recently retraced my steps and found that the magazines and cookbooks are much more user friendly now in 2016 than when I began in 1997. The diabetic books and magazines do not have desserts on the cover as much as when I started looking at those in 2009. I flipped through the books and found there were still fancy ingredients that were supposed to be better. Here is a sample:

Ahi tuna, 50 cents per ounce, about $6.00 a steak

Fennel bulb, not available in my neighborhood

Chia seed, 90.5 cents an ounce

Flax oil, $1.08 per ounce

Probiotics, 56.88 cents per ounce

Real maple syrup, 91.53 cents per ounce

Coconut oil, 50 cents per ounce

Saffron, $410.50 per ounce

These were ingredients in actual recipes I found. To be fair, that quantity of saffron would only be found in high end restaurants but the home package runs around $20, which is more than many people can afford who need to eat heathy the most. It is no wonder my students were so discouraged. It's no wonder they and I chose things like:

Bagged sugar frosted cereal, 9 cents an ounce

Soda, 2 cents an ounce

Macaroni and cheese mix, as low as 27 cents a box

It appeared to be cheaper, much cheaper.

I know these people who write these programs are well intentioned and some have really good research and ideas. They obviously live at a much higher income level than myself (even at the height of my career) or perhaps you do. The closest I got to this was an exercise expert saying that rice and beans are very healthy and it can be done. She gave no further ideas on the television program that day. I had one meal idea. I needed more. Healthy living appeared to be for the rich in this country. I searched some more.

In the textbook I used to teach the wellness class, it identified the two best oils for health eating: canola and olive. I priced them at the store too:

Olive oil, 3 cents per ounce and

Canola oil, 5 cents per ounce

Okay, now I was getting somewhere. I could buy it in small bottles. I traded whole milk for 2% and then to skim. The food fads went through what was essential to healthy eating by eliminating fats, carbohydrates, or protein one at a time. I knew it was all wrong to do it. It was essential to have all three as it said in the textbook. Always. Then different food items were chosen as the "bad" foods like eggs and milk. Substitutes were put on the market. Since then science has changed their minds. Real eggs always taste better than the substitute or just egg whites. Milk substitutes are very helpful for those with lactose intolerance and are tasty too. I even found some at the dollar store. I particularly do not have any reaction to milk so I drink skim.

Then I got the diagnosis of Prediabetes in 2009 after eating four lemon filled doughnuts one right after another. I had unknowingly given myself a glucose test by eating those doughnuts and I had a similar reaction to an actual glucose test when I was pregnant with my first child, at the doctor's office. I was nervous and anxious as my blood sugar climbed and then crashed. I felt terrible. I went to the doctor and she took a blood test. My morning fasting blood sugar was 109, Prediabetes.

"You are lucky," she said. "Many people don't know until it is much later on. How did you know?" I told her it felt similar to the test when I was diagnosed with Gestational Diabetes years before. (I was diabetic with both pregnancies and followed a food plan.)

She gave me a diet that had a calorie count limit and foods not to eat. I couldn't make that work either. I felt crummy for a long while. I found that orange juice should be kept on hand for when the blood sugar is low. I drank too much of it. I found I was very sensitive to orange juice in regulating my blood sugar. I stopped drinking it. I found some diabetic recipes in cookbooks and magazines. The cooking was so labor intensive and there were not many recipes that tasted good. The books were loaded with adapted sweets recipes in an effort for people to not be deprived. I did not want to live my life like this. I settled on *Cooking Light Magazine* as a compromise and started exercising.

I still had the handouts my doctor had given me and looked them over recently. It was by a diabetes drug manufacturing company. They had several items on it I found questionable. They had bread, crackers, flour tortillas, rice, pasta, bagel, and corn chips in the starch group. There was a sample meal plan that included artificially sweetened hot cocoa mix on it. They included potatoes as a starchy vegetable. There was juice included. There was sausage, pork spare ribs, cutlets, and wieners included too, all processed foods. It also allowed whipped topping. I have come to know that white flour version breads or the high fat meats or whipped topping they listed could be eaten occasionally but I didn't know there was something better, much better waiting in the literature for me. There was no mention of whole grains. There was no mention of sodium or sugar limits. They weren't specific enough in their guidelines. It was no wonder I abandoned this handout printed in 2001. My blood sugar reading indicated it wasn't working. I decided to go online and see what the company who wrote it and others like it suggest now. Most of the ones I looked at did no more than suggest the medications for diabetes be part of a healthy diet and exercise. That's it. Some also had links to the American Diabetes Association. The medical field appears to have learned a lot between 2001 and 2016.

During that time too I learned that type 2 prediabetes can be reversed or delayed. I was major surprised when I heard that. It made my search for the answer that much more focused. I would find out. I would. As I looked, I decided to exercise.

I got up off the couch. It felt crummy to exercise as I began. I had all kind of sensations I did not like during and after exercise. My fingertips swelled. I had to use the restroom frequently. I would feel hot and cold. I would be so exhausted afterwards I took and nap and was very tired the rest of the day. I pushed on when I heard it was not the body but the mind that is the problem at this point. Sure felt like my body. I pushed on and surprised myself.

I water walked in the swimming pool back and forth until I was strong enough to swim. I took up yoga with a video and then went to a yoga studio for classes. I walked laps at the mall. I became a member of a gym and swam every day and sat in the hot tub afterwards. I loved the hot tub. I moved and the gym near me had no pool. I quit. The blaring music bothered me and all the TV screens playing sometimes horrible things. It made no sense to me that exercising at a gym would fix one part of my health and disturb another. I wanted to quit the gym but didn't know what to do. I liked outside but I let the weather be the excuse. It can get very hot in Houston.

I collected recipes that were healthier versions of my favorite foods. I took care of myself best when I was on vacation. My work schedule didn't permit me to exercise outside of work so I exercised midpoint during my day which was at 3pm. They didn't like it. I asked for permission to do it and got "no" for an answer when clearly others got "yes". I saw a friend riding his bicycle in the neighborhood and took up walking outside. Quite by accident I discovered a wonderful greenspace to walk. Even as a morning person this did not appeal to me until then. I walked because I liked him.

It was way different walking outside than walking in the mall I had done earlier. My first walk was around the block. It felt terrible. Over time, I worked up to walking a 5K, 3.1 miles, every day. I even participated in a 5K that was not just for runners. I could walk in the "race".

People go on and on about the benefits of exercise. I didn't get it. It sounded so much like just talk until the day I did an experiment with myself at the gym back when I was swimming. I ate lunch before I swam laps as recommended in the programs I tried, to have something to burn. I got to the gym and put on my swim suit. I took my blood sugar. I swam for about 30 minutes without stopping. When I was back in the locker room and dressed I took my blood sugar again. The drop was so dramatic it astounded me. I exercised as often as I could after that. Exercise became important and better than any medicine for me that day.

Finding the right foods to eat was still a puzzle. I learned the food pyramid and then my plate. The same one as on choosemyplate.gov by the US Department of Agriculture. It was in the textbook of the course I taught. I tried things a little at a time. I absolutely hated cooking at the end of a busy day. I went out to eat or picked up some prepared food from the grocery store.

I took a free class on Coursera "Cooking for Kids" for professional development that was work related. It is an online class by Maya Adam, a doctor who got Stanford University to add a class on heathy eating as a graduation requirement. It doesn't matter to her if any of us in the course had kids or not, she asks us to prepare food for at least one person ages 3-99. She explained that she too is busy as a medical doctor and three small boys under seven years old. She cooked every day. I realized that if she could do it, I could too. My life was much simpler at home than hers with my children grown. One of them was away at school the other was in and out with an active life. I cooked for my 19-year-old son. He became interested, much to my surprise as my former picky eater. We cooked together once a week. At the end of the course she uploaded most of the teaching videos on You Tube. I showed a few to my students.

When I worked I seemed to lose all I had gained from when I was on vacation. I blamed it on the schedule, demands of life, and responsibilities. Then I retired.

I had a choice when I retired to take care of myself or not. I had wanted to for so long and I had every excuse not to, like many. Now I had no excuses and less money. I couldn't eat out or buy convenience foods anymore. I couldn't afford to. So I cooked. The right conditions had come for me. I did this for three months. Then it was time to go to my annual check-up. My doctor looked at my weight and blood pressure. "What have you been doing?" She asked. I told her I retired and was taking care of myself. She said to keep going, whatever I was doing. She told me usually when people retire, it gets worse not better. She looked at my numbers from the year before. I think she fully expected to put me on some kind of medicine for type 2 diabetes. Days later when the blood work came back everything was normal with the exception of the triglycerides and the A1C both still needed a little work. She had hopes what I was doing would take care of it.

I finally hit on the one thing that made all the difference:

Fresh food is better than processed food. It makes a big difference to go from processed to all fresh foods. My numbers proved it.

I got the idea from Dr. Maya Adam who stressed we must cook and not eat processed foods. It took my own experimenting with it for it to become real to me. She meant no processed food at all.

She was clearly cooking with organic food from a high end grocery, I had been to such stores on little trips to look at what eating healthy looked like. I knew I couldn't afford those foods. So I did the next best thing, I bought the same foods as what she had, only the conventional ones and were in season and on sale. It worked! Next thing I knew I was craving things like mushrooms, beets, and berries instead of processed and fast foods.

Several weeks in, I decided I wanted a hamburger from a fast food restaurant that was a favorite. I was surprised how flavorless it tasted, how it didn't satisfy, and it messed up my system for the evening at so drastic a change.

I felt better eating fresh foods. It was good to be satisfied and know that my blood work showed it. I had finally found what I needed from resources that are free.

The one other thing I learned from the fitness folks is this: always keep moving.

I take breaks in my day to exercise and generally move about. I feel better when I do.

I have a new "trainer" too. My little grandson is on the move and when I care for him a couple of days a week it means I have to lift him, play with him on the floor and get back up. We dance to music with me holding him. He loves unrolling the yoga mat and crawling under me doing downward facing dog. That came about when he was doing an invented crawl of his own and often went into a downward facing dog position. I rolled out the mat and joined him. He laughed. Now we do yoga together. We go for walks in the stroller several times a day in an effort to calm him and change things up. He is a relentless "trainer" I can't say no to. We are having the time of our lives.

This I know: any program without both the healthy eating and exercise is no program at all.

My appetite also seemed to diminish when I did the things I loved to do. I got caught in the moment doing these things and it lead to me not grazing all day like I had been. It was satisfying in a different way that eating didn't fulfill. I felt I was on to something for myself. I put the scale in the cabinet and threw out my alarm clock. I decided to live on "Susan Time" rather than the whims and expectations of others. It was both surprisingly freeing and scary. It worked for me because I am a self-starter and can invent things for myself. I had been spending my work vacations trying to figure out how to fill the expansive time I was anticipating for myself. It helped me get the results I did.

What I Ate Before

I have this notebook of old menus. I put it together because I could never remember what I liked to eat when it came time to make a shopping list. The notebook became a place to keep them after I went shopping and the menu was through for the week. I used it as a reference for more recipe ideas as I planned my week and later for this book. What I found was my eating habits had changed a lot over time. The next morning, I decided to take a closer look at what I ate for the 35 random weeks I managed to keep the menus and get it into the notebook. The menus were made sometime between 2000-2013. There were also 6 lists I had made of food ideas that I could make future menus from. It was meant to be for reference. What I found was a time capsule of my eating when I thought I was doing okay with eating healthy these particular weeks. My intention was to give myself a variety of foods I liked. It seemed that if I didn't do this than I had the tendency to cook the same thing all the time. When I looked at them in April of 2016 I was horrified at what I found.

Here are the results:

There were 305 food items that included a mix of ingredients, sandwiches, entrees, snack foods, and desserts. Out of the 305 food items I made only 107 healthy choices. I couldn't believe it. That was only about 35% of the foods I bought. I know too I didn't eat them all. There was a lot of food waste, especially of the fruits and vegetables I bought. That means 65% of what I bought was a bad choice.

Here is the breakdown of my bad choices:

12% were processed foods

15% were foods made mostly with white flour

13% were foods with high sugar/white sugar content

5% were foods made with white potatoes

6% were food made with white rice as most of the dish

14% were high fat foods

All of the above fatty food contributed daily to my blood sugar reading for the day.

My healthy food choices were equally as surprising:

35% were proteins (lean meats, beans, and meat substitutes)

31% were vegetables

11% were fruits

9% were tomato based foods

8% were whole grains

1% were healthy fats

2% were snacks, desserts, and condiments

That meant only 13% of my total diet was fruits and vegetables. No wonder I got the diagnoses of Prediabetes. I really was still searching for the answer. I knew that then.

Of the bad choices, the foods appeared to be good choices. When I bought the processed chicken pieces and broke them open there was white breast meat inside. There was tomato based foods that was recommended as having fewer calories that was recommended by one of the programs I participated in. I bought the meats in packages that appeared to be sliced off a bigger roast. I bought items that would save me time. I had no idea the bread products were such a big part of my diet. I craved them constantly and sugary foods too. I didn't know about the impact of white flour, rice, and white potatoes on my blood sugar. I thought if I added more vegetables to these dishes, I would be okay. I don't remember what I thought about the high fat foods. Eating seemed to be a mine field then. I could not stop eating until I found out. It just doesn't work that way.

Of the good choices, the foods that I chose were sometimes not that appealing. I steamed the vegetables in the microwave, they came packed to just put them in and set the timer. They didn't taste like much. I ate a lot of salad and raw vegetables to the point it felt like grazing. (Some called it "Rabbit Food", jokingly, of course. I felt like a rabbit sometimes.) There had to be better recipes for me so I searched for some and found a few I liked. These recipes were not on the menus. The fruits I ate whole like snack foods. I prepared quite a lot of tomato based entrees from scratch. The whole grains were in the form of healthy breakfast cereal and granola in bars and loose in bags. Interestingly, my healthier meals were centered around meat and too big a portion of it.

One thing that the menus does not really reveal is how often I really ate the foods. The menus were the plan and apparently not that good of one. I remember eating out a lot too, especially Mexican, Italian, and Chinese foods (all Americanized versions of really good food I have never eaten). Then there was fast food, too frequent to count, that I ate in the car to some seemingly important thing I had to do.

What I Eat Now

I looked over my cash register grocery receipts and determined I bought and ate about 243 servings of food this month. Of those servings I ate:

5.7% White flour products

2.4% fatty proteins

1.6% snacks and deserts

.8% less healthy fats but no trans fats

This totals 12.9% less healthy foods for the month.

The healthy choices for the month were as follows:

12.7% lean proteins (lean meats, beans, and meat substitutes)

17.2% fresh vegetables

12.3% fresh fruits, including 1 can fruit in juice and 4 servings 100% fruit juice with no sugar added

1.6% tomato based sauces

25.5% whole grains

.8% healthy fats

1.6% Snacks and desserts

16.4% dairy, most of it skim milk

The total of Healthy food choices was 87.1% for the month. The results are dramatic at first glance. Let me take a closer look at the two time periods.

Comparison

Below is the comparison for my unhealthy food choices:

12% were processed foods before and 0% now.

15% were foods made mostly with white flour before and 5.7% white flour products now.

13% were foods with high sugar/white sugar content and 1.6% snacks and deserts now.

5% were foods made with white potatoes and 0% white potatoes now.

6% were food made with white rice as most of the dish and the rice was included with the white grains and is .8%.

14% were high fat foods and now it is .8% less healthy fats but no trans fats.

My unhealthy eating habits are down 55.1% and my blood sugar is normal.

Below is the comparison of my healthy food choices:

35% were proteins (lean meats, beans, and meat substitutes) and are 12.7% proteins (lean meats, beans, and meat substitutes).

31% were vegetables and now are 17.2% fresh vegetables.

11% were fruits and now are 12.3% fresh fruits, including 1 can fruit in juice and 4 servings 100% fruit juice with no sugar added.

9% were tomato based foods and are now 1.6% tomato based sauces.

8% were whole grains and now are 25.5% whole grains.

1% were healthy fats and now are .8% healthy fats.

2% were snacks, desserts, and condiments and are now 1.6% Snacks and desserts.

There is no record for dairy in my before report. I bought them but they were not on my menus now they are 16.4% dairy, most of it skim milk.

The results are surprising here too. Although I am eating 22.3% meat, 1.3% more fruit, I am eating less vegetables and more whole grains. The whole grains are good but it would be a place to improve with less whole grains and more vegetables. As for the tomato based products, it is okay to substitute other vegetables for them. It is not a necessary component of a healthy diet. "Eat a rainbow" is the recommendation for choosing vegetables. Dairy for someone my age and weight is 2 serving a day so I am over by 4 servings for the month, not a big difference. The fats and the snacks were about the same. I don't think that needs changing. I used canola oil and olive oil back then too. The lack of enough vegetables could be the very reason my LDL numbers are not quite normal yet.

To improve, I think if I got a diagram of "my plate" and how they divide it up posted in my kitchen where I serve my plate, I think I would do even better with getting more vegetables without measuring.

Health Reports

I have been keeping my health reports sporadically over time. Here is a glimpse:

<u>2009</u>

Blood Glucose 108 (should be less than 100)

Total Cholesterol: 182 (should be less than 200)

Triglycerides: 175 (should be less than 150)

HDL (good cholesterol): 45 (should be more than 50)

LDL (bad cholesterol): 102 (Should be less than 130)

<u>Blood Sugar Journal I kept:</u>

2011-2015 All morning blood tests over 100 from 108-176. Mostly hovered around 108-120, two tests below 100, two tests above 150. All blood tests were done at home first thing in the morning before eating using a Sidekick blood glucose testing system and separate store brand lancets and pen. Below is a sample.

<u>2011</u>

December 7, 2011 weight 193.8, blood sugar 110

<u>2012</u>

January 1, 2012 weight 192.9, blood sugar 113

June 15, 2012 weight 198.1, blood sugar 104

September 24, 2012 weight 188.2, blood sugar 108

<u>2013</u>

February 2, 2013 weight 192, blood sugar 109

<u>2016</u>

April 26, 2016 weight 187 blood sugar 94

May 13, 2016 weight 188.1. blood sugar 94

May 30, 2016 weight 183.9 and blood sugar 104

<u>Conclusion</u>: Though a lot of emphasis is put on weight loss in managing the blood sugar, having a continuous supply of fresh fruits and vegetables is essential. The May 30, 2016 week I ran out of fruits and vegetables and it took its toll. A few days prior my blood sugar was 114. I exercised and lost weight that week too. This is not as simple as one might think. Vegetables matter.

Foods I Buy and Eat

So let's get down to it. What exactly am I eating? Here is the list of what I have eaten from November-April. The good news is some recipes I used are included too. I have seen such lists and not really know what to do with it.

Vegetables:

winter squashes (acorn, butternut), sweet potatoes, onions, carrots, parsnips, beets, cabbage, cauliflower, broccoli, spinach, red cabbage, mushrooms, tomatoes, bell pepper (green, red, orange, yellow), green beans, celery, cucumber, asparagus, eggplant, Brussels sprouts, tomatillos, poblamo peppers

Note: I buy only the fresh firm vegetables. I find out when they put them out for sale and buy those days. The in season vegetables will be on sale and are in the circular I get in the mail.

Fruits:

apples, citrus fruits (lemon, orange, lime), berries (strawberries, blueberries, raspberries), bananas, cantaloupe

Note: Same directions as the vegetables.

Breads and Grains:

Sourdough bread, whole wheat tortillas, corn tortillas, whole wheat cereals, pancake mixes without white flour, popcorn, graham crackers, oat granola bars, rolled oats, bread crumbs

Note: I learned that sourdough bread is the only white bread Prediabetics can have years ago. It seems that the American Diabetes Association has changed their stance on the foods that can be eaten and now include all foods in the right portions.

Choose myplate suggests more whole grains in addition to the white. Changing from white flour products to whole wheat is quite a change. Some products have half white and half wheat in them, a step I took to learn to eat the whole wheat products. I buy whole kernel popcorn, not microwaveable, to control the amount of salt and the kind of fat I cook it in. I don't buy any wheat bread that has molasses in it. They use the molasses (sugar syrup) to color white bread. WIC doesn't choose this bread on their list for pregnant women. Their labels are a help to choosing healthy foods, I have found. I learned too recently that both white and whole grains effect the blood sugar the same. That came as quite a surprise and I am now being more careful of my bread intake.

Healthy Fats:

Avocado, raw nuts, olive oil, canola oils

Note: The raw nuts that are priced the lowest are found in the baking aisle of the grocery store. The oils can be purchased in small quantities. I do not buy "vegetable" oil, it is a mix of oils that are not just these nutritious oils but a blend of various oils.

Dairy:

Yogurt, cheeses (mozzarella, Colby), cottage cheese, butter or margarine in small amounts, crema, skim milk

Note: I buy cheeses in blocks and cut them up into smaller portions. I freeze some of the portions so I don't eat it all at once. I grate it myself over foods, never enough to be gloppy or stringy. Crema is Mexican style cream similar to sour cream. The butter/margarine debate is quite hot right now. A very small amount of real butter in foods can add flavor that margarine cannot. It is very high in saturated fat so very small amounts are recommended. Yet the margarine is very spreadable and made of oil. The good ones are the ones that become liquid at room temperature.

Proteins:

Lean chicken tenderloins and skinless chicken thighs, lean boneless pork chops, fish fillets (tilapia, salmon, flounder), shrimp, dried beans, raw nuts (almonds, walnuts, sunflower seeds), peanut butter, eggs, cheese, ground turkey, hummus, tuna (packed in water)

Note: These lesser quality cuts of meat can be purchased in larger packages either fresh or frozen, most peanut butter has shortening in it and the healthier version would be at the peanut butter machine in the grocery store where I can grind it fresh from the nuts in the machine. I get to choose the quantity I want, and it is sold by weight. I don't eat much beef these days as the lowest fat ground beef is high priced.

Seasonings:

Garlic, black pepper, herbs (fresh or dried, basil, sage, cilantro, cumin, ginger, nutmeg, pumpkin pie spice), citrus fruits, seasoning mixes, chilies (mild canned, fresh), cinnamon

Sauces:

Tomato sauce (Italian style), Stir fry sauce, soy sauce, Tikka Masala sauce, Salsas (green and red)

Occasionally:

White flour, white rice, white pasta, white potato, watermelon, 100% fruit juices with no high fructose corn syrup, sweets (cake, pie, candy, ice cream), French bread, bolillo rolls, mini bagels, maple syrup (with no high fructose corn syrup), honey, fruit jam, turkey bacon, chocolate

Note: I do use these items in cooking sometimes and for flavor. I don't want to feel deprived of the things I like.

Note: There are so many other great healthy food choices that I don't particularly know how to cook or haven't eaten before not on this list. Some are expensive because of where I live. I made the list to reflect my tastes, part of the country I live, and my culture.

Note: I did not include iceberg lettuce because although it is not harmful, it doesn't offer as much nutrition as so many other dark leafy greens. I don't buy it for that reason.

Cost

I promised $176 a month in my title of this book. How did it come to cost so little to buy healthy food? For the first three months I went into my bank account and added up the cost from all the places I shop for food from November to January. It came to an average of $288 a month. The first month was a move to a new place to live and it ran higher to start over and stock the kitchen about $350. The next month was about $288. The third month dipped low, about $170. I didn't think it could actually go that low and there might be a mistake. The fourth and fifth months I didn't keep track. The sixth month, April, I kept the receipts and added up only the food when I realized that I had other expenses in there too like nonfood items and cat care items. The total for that month was $176.11. Probably the most accurate cost after being established on my new place. Just to be sure, the receipts for May totaled $170.01.

So as you can see, it took a little time to learn to be frugal in my approach to food. The waste is very low, about 5 items for the 5 months. One of which I bought bad and didn't know it. That is easy to do in discount type stores that sell more than grocery items. They don't keep up with it as closely.

I didn't deprive myself either, I eat what I used to buy in the restaurants: Mexican food, Italian food, Chinese Food, and Indian food. I learned to make my favorite dishes I used to always order when I went out. It has been kind of an adventure that way.

As for the tempting foods like sweets and desserts, I haven't eaten that much of them since I buy in small quantities. I can go several days now without dessert at all. It keeps the cost down to limit the sweets, a craving of mine, apparently.

A Program of My Own

As I reflect on this "plan" I follow and made up for myself I took in consideration a number of things. They are as follows:

The kind of foods I like to eat

My culinary skill

The amount of time I wanted to spend cooking each day

My health needs

The places I have available to shop for food and to exercise

The nutritional information I had

The time I set aside to figure out what is best and works for me

What I love to do and how to spend my time

My food budget

Resources available to help me

Where I live in the US

My culture

My food memories

How my family traditions and holidays are celebrated

There are probably more things I took in consideration too. I have no problem with this not working for anyone but me. It is the story that matters really. That it can be done. Anyone can do the thing that matters to them and to live a full and healthy life, if they set their mind to it.

Unfortunately, it was and is not easy. It was time consuming and I made a lot of mistakes. Although I know that some will follow this and get results as their plan too, I hope really it is a place to begin for a personal food journey people will tailor to themselves including the foods they like and consider their own health needs.

It was not easier for me to follow someone else's plan. Every one of them were not something I could sustain over time and become my way of life. I couldn't measure, count, and weigh my food every day and call it a life. I couldn't obsess over the way I looked and foods I "couldn't" eat. I couldn't live for weigh ins or weigh myself every time I went by my scale. I had to find a way to be me and let food become a natural part of life again. I found that through doing what I loved to do. It made for a beautiful way to spend my time.

I can't really say about how doing what I loved made all that obsessing clear up. I just put all of it in place as I began my creative life in retirement. I would not say I gained happiness either. I gained me. Instead of 5 minutes of the day for myself, that I had back in1997. I now have 95% of the day doing what I love to do in 2016. The rest was stuff I don't like, namely, house cleaning and paperwork.

I am not the first one to do this either. An interesting read is titled "The Writing Diet" by Julia Cameron. She found that she and others lost weight as they tune into what they loved to do too. It was indeed surprising for me too to discover my clothes loosen as I did what I loved and made doing what I loved a priority.

Maybe it is a form of truth telling that I hadn't explored yet. In my world there are not that many introspective type people. I think I am on to something here so I thought I would share it to the three people who could benefit. So onward we go, it is good to start somewhere then not at all.

Getting Started

Making choices of heathy foods was a lot of work at first. It is surprising how habitual food shopping can be. Here are the food categories I choose from:

Lean meats

Fruits

Vegetables

Proteins (includes beans, eggs, dairy, nuts)

Breads and Grains

The choice of store will either make it easier or harder to shop healthy. They tend to feature impulse items on the ends of the aisles. The lower end stores will have much more less healthy foods to walk by but the healthy choices are there if you go with the expectation to find them and have a list. The higher end store will have higher quality less healthy foods to walk past too that are expensive. Both are hard to do. It is best to have a list and not browse. It is best to not shop hungry.

Let's go shopping...

Step one: make a menu and shopping list. Don't go to the store hungry.

Step two: add up the items as you choose the items. I round up the price and keep a running total across the top of my list. For example, if eggs are $3.50 I will write 4 at the top of the page. If the next item is half gallon of milk and is $1.97 I will cross out the 4 and write 6. That keeps a running total and is usually less at the register from all the rounding up. When things are particularly tight I go to the self-serve register and can leave items behind without embarrassing myself in front of a cashier to take items off the total.

Step three: Comparison shop. Look at the price per serving as a better guide than the total price. Sometimes organic foods cost less than conventional. Get them when they are the better buy, of course. Get items that help to portion control. Surprisingly, the Dollar Store is good at this. Sometimes they are more per serving but if you know you are tempted to eat the whole package in one sitting like say, chips, a small is a better choice than a large one for your health.

Buy already prepared sauces to give your foods flavor. Many times, to buy the ingredients to make the sauce would cost more than getting the sauce already prepared. Examples are stir fry sauces, BBQ, dressings, and tomato based sauces.

Step four: pay for it using store discount cards to give you discounts on specials. I don't use coupons because I have never seen one on the kinds to foods that really matter on a healthy diet like carrots, bell peppers, and lean meats.

Step five: Divide up lean meats in portion sizes for the freezer and wrap them up for later in the week. Put all the food away.

I really don't like to cook. There I said it. I don't like how it can take over the day. I searched high and low and learned to stream line it. The crock pot is one of my favorites for this. I love how you dump everything it in and walk away from it. A few hours later, a wonderful aroma that something is cooking is in the air while I worked on a project, went for a walk or took a nap.

If you don't know how to cook, then it is time to learn. Maya Adam's videos are really good as she is a home cook and keeps it simple, unlike the food TV channels. I knew how to cook and found the videos interesting to see how to cook healthy using the best techniques. For me it was a refresher.

Chop up everything before you turn on the heat. The largest knife is your friend. It is the work horse of the kitchen. You can use separate chopping boards for meat and vegetables or wash a plastic one thoroughly between uses. Same with the knife. This is for food safety to keep you from making yourself sick.

Make yourself a nice plate of food with a variety of textures and colors. The guide is this: "eat a rainbow" of colors of produce. It is not only pretty and appealing but it is well balanced. Use the choose my plate guide on how much to put on your plate. Big servings of meat and bread are out for a healthy diet for me.

I found that there was information on serving sizes in terms of your own handful. There is an idea out there that your serving sizes are what your own hand will hold, if you have to measure. I incorporated it into the recipes in this book.

When you first begin, it may be a surprise to find how filling these foods are compared to the processed ones. A sweet potato cut up and oven roasted into "fries" will be more satisfying than a whole bag of potato chips. I eventually ate less food when I am routinely satisfied and exercise every day.

Mixed foods are something that some people love such as casserole types and one dish meals. These are very hard to determine what is in it if you don't make it yourself and can control the sodium and fat. Canned soup based recipes are out, tomato and broth based recipes are in for me, though I love them so much and was raised on some of this type of food. When I do, I double up on the vegetables and less on the starches like rice and pasta. My blood sugar reading never lies the next day. That is where the truth is told, for me.

It's not the food sometimes but what you do it that makes it healthier or not. Canola oil is good to sauté with and stir fry. The oil itself doesn't change it. The amount of it in the food does. It is possible to take something healthy and overdo it by using too much oil, cooking the flavor out, immersing it in too much sauce, and/or eating too much of it at once.

I looked into the healthy types of cooking: roasting, grilling, stewing, steaming, sautéing, and stir frying are the healthier ones. Deep frying, wrapping things in dough, immersing them in gravy, or pouring dressings, sugar, or heavy cream sauces are the less healthy types of cooking I tend to avoid. These methods start with great food and overwhelm it with calories of the other. Keeping the food as close to how to bought it is best for me and recommended by professionals.

The next section are recipes based on the ideas I have just mentioned. Know too there are more online to find now that you know what to look for. Eating should still be a pleasure.

Free Resources

Free website: choosemyplate.gov

Free course on Coursera: Child Nutrition and Cooking by Dr. Maya Adam

You Tube: Dr. Maya Adam

TED Talks: Dr. Maya Adam "Why We Fight with Our Food"

Another favorite:

TED Talks: Jamie Oliver "Teach Every Child About Food"

Now all my recipe finding made sense and what I was to do.

◊◊◊

A Bit of Humor: "The Whole Thing..."

There was this television commercial in 1972 for Alka Seltzer where a man sits in the edge of the bed at night repeating the sentence, "I can't believe I ate the whole thing." The solution was to take Alka Seltzer for an upset stomach. Over eating was regretful and it became okay to talk about it openly in 1972. So one day, this idea came to class through one of my students, who wanted to know about controlling the urge to eat the whole package of something. My response surprised her.

"How about a whole box of strawberries instead?" She was shocked to get that answer. She and a few others talked about how they couldn't. I told them I did. It wasn't enough of an answer for them. I didn't go further with it and went on with the next topic.

I ate out quite a lot then, about five nights a week maybe even every day. I decided to notice how fruits and vegetables were served when I went out to eat. It turned out to be quite sparingly, even as little as a garnish on a plate. A really good restaurant with lots of vegetables and fruits was hard to find. No wonder it was so surprising to get that answer.

So let me introduced the idea that it is okay to eat the whole box of strawberries, a whole cantaloupe, or mushrooms if you want. They will be packed full of nutrition the bag or box of the regretful foods will never have and likely be cheaper too. Here are the numbers, in Houston, of course:

A bag of chips is $2.99.

A whole cantaloupe in season is 99 cents.

A whole box of strawberries is $2.50.

I think it is okay to indulge a little on real food. Really I do. Perhaps it is cultural and socially acceptable to complain about it too.

Real food is good, tasty, and filling. No Alka Seltzer needed.

Frequently Asked Questions

What are processed foods?

These are foods that are cooked at a factory and shipped to the grocery store for convenience. Examples of these foods are: frozen dinners, frozen pizza, frozen fried meats, crackers, chips, cookies. They are usually high in salt or sugar. Canned foods can also be processed like soups, noodle meals, fruits packed in syrup, vegetables packed with high sodium. Some of these foods are also prepared at the grocery store for convenience. They have labeling to let you know the sugar and salt content. For a complete list of the unhealthy choices I made, you can find it in the back of this book in the "Things I learned along the way" section.

Do you measure your food?

No. I learned by the look of it from my dieting experiences and search. The myplate diagram is enough to determine portion sizes with the right sized plate they recommend. I admit I was extremely hungry at first when learning portion sizes in one of the programs I participated in and adapting to them from eating more than double what I should. I had support of a program for when I did this the first time. It was very hard to both cut back and start moving.

Do you work out?

To me, working out involves planning and a variety of activities like strength training and cardio and someone measuring it. In that regard, then no. I exercise every day. Usually walking. No power walking. No cute walking suits. No electronic devices strapped to me. No fancy shoes, just the ones I got on sale. I mosey at about 2.5 miles per hour. Honest. Everyone passes me up, everyone. Sometimes yoga, which is strength training that helps with balance. Sometimes swimming, just because I like water. Sometimes caring for my grandson.

Did you lose weight?

Yes, 15 pounds but it wasn't intentional. Once I found that out and started stepping on the scale, I would gain some back. When I took my focus off the scale it got better. I could tell my clothes felt looser. My doctor scrolled back to my heaviest until now and I had lost 27 pounds. There were some ups and downs, be assured.

Have you struggled with weight your whole life?

No, I was normal weight and active as a child. I rode my bike, swam, and walked. It became a struggle in my adult years before I had children and got worse.

How do you manage portion control?

Doing what I love has a lot to do the rest of the day and exercise has a lot of effect on my food intake. I don't have the crazy cravings to eat all the time when I do what I love. I don't really snack much when I have a great project to work on. When I walk a 5K I am not that hungry afterwards. The cool thing is I am not "white knuckling it" with willpower. I make a good healthy plate and eat. Seconds are not as often as before.

No willpower?

Not as much as it was before. To me, willpower is needed when a person really doesn't want to do something. This I do want to do. I love the foods I make for myself. They taste good and satisfy me. When I find I need will power is when I feel stressed about something and it is time to reset my priorities to what I love to do instead of obsessing over things like how much I am eating. I don't really do that as much anymore either.

What beverages do you drink?

Water, water with lemon or lime slices, herbal tea, decaf tea, regular tea. For a treat I like a root beer, lemonade or a Chai Tea Latte, a passion tea lemonade with half sweetener at Starbucks. It is hard to drink something with such a high sugar content after working so hard. I know it will show up in my blood monitoring in the morning.

What about GMO's and the healthier organic foods?

Some will argue about GMOs and organic produce. I don't know much about that. As I see it, if I eat processed foods I get in trouble with my blood sugar. Real food is best for me. I ate all conventional middle range produce, 50% whole grains, skim dairy products, and lean meats suggested on my plate for the numbers I got. I bought what I could afford.

What about microwaving healthy foods?

I can't afford those healthy microwaveable foods. I recently moved and they didn't provide a microwave where I live. I was offered one from family and didn't take it. It is too tempting to buy the foods I shouldn't when I have a microwave. The food I make cooks in about the same amount of time it takes to drive down to the nearest fast food restaurant, eat, and drive home. It also makes my home smell good and homey. They taste much better. Even my daughter who finished certification in culinary arts and is a chef at a local restaurant agreed with me that my cooking is improving. Dr. Maya Adam doesn't appear to eat them either.

What methods do you use without a microwave?

I am big into cooking in parchment or foil packs, stir fried foods, sautéed foods, skillet meals, oven roasted, crock pot, and one pot meals. I never deep fry or use high sodium foods like most canned foods have.

What else did you learn from Dr. Maya Adam?

To never use spray oils. She doesn't like the propellant in them. I experimented with pouring oil in a sauté pan and rubbing it around with paper towel. It soaks up too much of the oil and foods stick that way. I discovered that just a little oil in a cup with a pastry brush works better and my pans seem better too.

Do you buy in quantity?

I don't stock up on foods unless the weather is going to be really bad. I buy a few days at a time. My refrigerator goes nearly empty frequently. This keeps waste to a minimum.

Do you watch TV while you eat?

The TV plays music while I eat. It is important to pay attention while I eat and enjoy the healthy food I made for myself.

Where do you shop?

The grocery store is a half a block away I can walk to. The dollar store that is a little over a half a block away in the other direction I walk to. I buy the cheapest for the money including store brand and WIC foods. Though I do not qualify for WIC, the foods they choose are super healthy and marked with labels in the store for easy shopping.

They have healthy foods at the dollar store?

Yes, I found popcorn seeds, dill pickles, frozen berries, mayonnaise, strawberry jam, crackers, pasta, tomato sauce, tuna packed in water, salmon, spices, and dried beans. Another visit I found teriyaki marinade, rolled oats, country style mustard, chickpeas, turkey burgers, graham crackers, Worcestershire sauce, and canned pineapple. I was surprised too. The dollar store sometimes carries name brands. The other brands are comparable to the grocery store brands. The small packaging is great for portion control and providing more variety on a tight budget. The availability changes at the store I go to. It makes it real hard to plan a menu, so I go there first at the beginning of the month.

What about spoiling foods? Don't fresh foods spoil fast?

Yes, they do. That is the reason I buy in small quantities. I freeze the lean meats and cheeses in portions to cook later. I buy the vegetables and fruits that naturally have a longer shelf life than others. I don't eat salad much at all. I ate a lot of salad when on those food programs I could not stick with. I would rather have a hot meal these days.

What are the healthy long shelf life foods you suggested?

Some vegetables last longer than others. These were foods our foremothers grew to keep over the winter in the root cellar where the temperature remained cool. These vegetables are: winter squashes, sweet potatoes, onions, carrots, parsnips, beets, apples, citrus fruits, cabbage. Cauliflower and broccoli will also last longer than some other produce. These should last a whole week in the refrigerator, maybe longer. When I started to try and eat healthy years ago I bought a lot of lettuce and berries that spoiled quickly. It was expensive to keep these as they spoiled before the week was through. It felt like wasted money, which it was.

How many meals do you eat a day?

Three. Breakfast. Lunch. Dinner. One regular meal and two light meals, I learned this about myself while on a program. I move the regular sized meal around. Sometimes a snack. Sometimes a fruit dessert.

Are there any fresh foods you don't eat?

Yes, because I have Prediabetes I don't eat watermelon, orange juice, and white potatoes because they make my blood sugar spike. I usually treat juice, white flour products, and starchy vegetables as a once in a while treat. They also mess with my blood sugar. Funny, I know. Treats used to be cookies, candy, pies and cakes. I do eat a few modified desserts from time to time and all out cheat on the major holidays but not enough to make me sleepy.

Do you use the Diabetic Food Exchange system?

No, not at this point. It may be in my future. I am going to keep walking and eating this way as long as I can.

Do you have any other things that contributed to your weight problem?

Yes, being in the wrong environment that was too stressful and demanding for me. I didn't know how to choose what was right for me. I gave in to the demands and put myself last. That was the perfect combination for my health to decline and the weight went on.

Do you have any other resources to get me started?

Yes, I like *Cook Fresh* and *Clean Eating* magazines. I would recommend anything by the American Diabetes Association in regards to their books and website. I still like *Cooking Light* magazine and their books. I found too some new words that indicate really healthy eating "Superfoods" and "healing foods" which appear in book titles and magazine articles. The source tends to be a good one with these words in it. There is a huge emphasis on vegetables in these publications. Many of these resources can be found in your local public library for free.

Intrigued? Hope so. Let's begin.

Recipes

The recipes I have included are those I assemble the most often. Not lot of cooking happens. Yes, eating healthy can be low cost and quick. These are how I put together the healthy foods on the lists to suit me. I will not say that the foods are delicious, that is for you to decide and change to your own tastes. Food selections is funny like that.

Recipes for Breakfast

No Cook Fast breakfast 1
A variation of a breakfast I had at a hotel on a convention.

Yogurt, the kind I like (plain is better to add your own fruit)

Banana

Nuts, one handful

Open and eat. This is a very filling meal. I brought this to work for a quick lunch too.

No Cook Fast Breakfast 2
I had bagels the first time at a school I worked at.

2 mini bagels spread with cream cheese

 Whole in season fresh fruit

A handful of raw nuts

No Cook Breakfast 3

An old favorite with a protein as suggested by Dr. Maya Adam.

Cold cereal with milk and fruit.

A handful of raw nuts.

Fruit Cup and Yogurt

I had this at a hotel on convention.

2 or 3 fresh fruits cut up in a bowl

Vanilla yogurt

Sprinkle with granola cereal or broken granola bar, for crunch.

Sourdough English Muffin Sandwich

A variation of the popular restaurant breakfast.

1 English Muffin

1 egg

2 strips of Turkey Bacon or sautéed spinach with garlic, tomato, mushrooms and onion

A pat of healthy margarine or a teaspoon of canola oil

Toast English Muffin. In a sauté pan, melt the pat of butter or heat oil. Cut the turkey bacon and place in the pan. Cook until browned. Place aside turkey bacon pieces. For the vegetable variation sauté the vegetables first and leave in the pan. Break the egg into the pan, scramble the egg with the spatula. Cook egg through. Bacon bit left in the pan will go into the eggs giving it a campfire version of eggs. Place egg and bacon on half of the English muffin. Place the other half on top.

Omelet or Frittata with Vegetables

My own version that is a combination of restaurant and cookbook recipes.

Dice or finely slice the following vegetables:

¼ small onion

5 mushrooms

¼ bell pepper, orange

½ tomato

Sauté vegetables in a pan with olive oil. Cook until the vegetables are just cooked and still have their shape. Add:

Spinach, one handful, fresh prewashed

Let spinach cook down.

Add seasonings:

 Sea salt grinder, pepper grinder, garlic powder

Add:

2 or 3 beaten eggs

How you handle it from here will determine if you have a frittata or fancy scrambled eggs. If you move the whole mixture around, you have fancy scrambled eggs, if you don't you got a frittata. If you fold it over it is an omelet. The omelet needs to be cooked through so it is necessary to lift and let the egg mixture make contact with the pan until cooked through. The frittata just cooks through without moving it around.

Serve rolled up in a whole wheat tortilla or a Sourdough English Muffin on the side and slices of fresh fruit.

French Toast

A favorite as a child. I added the cinnamon. My daughter added the vanilla.

Beat together with a fork in a low dish:

1 egg

¼ cup of milk

A drop of vanilla

Heat a sauté pan with a pat of margarine or brushed with canola oil

Dip 1 slice of bread in the mixture

Sprinkle with cinnamon.

Place in the frying pan, cook until golden. Flip over. Sprinkle more cinnamon on the other side. Repeat with another slice of bread.

Spread with margarine and dribble with syrup.

Serve with whole fruit and turkey bacon.

Bran Muffins

Taken from the All-Bran Cereal Package. It is out of print and has been for quite a while. I increased the milk amount for a smoother texture muffin and lowered the baking temperature because of the dark pans and the more efficient ovens we have today.

In a bowl place:

2 Cups all Bran Cereal

1 1/2 Cups skim milk

Let sit until all the milk has been soaked up by the cereal.

Add:

1 egg

¼ cup of canola oil

Stir with a fork until smooth.

In another bowl place:

1 ¼ cup of flour

½ cup of sugar

1 Tablespoon baking powder

Blend with a fork. Pour into the cereal mixture. Mix until all dry ingredients are incorporated. Grease the muffin pan with a little canola oil and a pastry brush. Distribute the batter among the 12 wells of the pan. Bake at 350 degrees until a fork comes out clean, about 15 minutes.

Great warm or cold. Spread with margarine, if desired. Serve with cold skim milk or hot tea.

Pancakes

Another favorite as a child.

Whole wheat, oat, or mixed wheat pancake mix. Anything with no white flour.

Prepare as on the directions on box. Drizzle with maple syrup. Serve with fresh fruit on the side.

Grown up Oatmeal

A recipe that is a variation on a local restaurant.

Quick cooking Oatmeal

Fresh fruit, dried fruit, or canned fruit in juice

Raw nuts

Maple syrup

Cook according to directions on the box. Place in serving bowl. Place bite sized pieces of fruit on the top. Sprinkle with nuts. Top with a squeeze of maple syrup. Serve with milk.

Breakfast Tacos

I ate these the first time at a school in-service training.

2 eggs, scrambled

Vegetables of your choice (baby spinach, mushrooms, tomato, onion, garlic)

2 tortillas

Sauté the vegetables in canola oil. Add the scrambled eggs. Cook together eggs and vegetables. Spoon into tortillas.

Recipes for Lunch or Dinner

Chicken Enchiladas

A homemade version of my favorite restaurant dish.

Cook together in a small sauce pan over medium heat:

1 C bottled salsa verde, medium heat

2 or 3 fresh tomatillos with outer skins removed, diced

In a skillet place:

1 Tablespoon oil

3 chicken tenderloins, cut with kitchen shears

Cook chicken until golden and cooked through.

On a serving plate place:

2 corn tortillas

Place half the chicken on each tortilla

¼ cup salsa verde mixture

Sprinkle with: grated Colby cheese

1 tablespoon of crema, divided among the tortillas for the authentic taste

Roll up each tortilla with the contents inside. Top with the remaining salsa verde, more Colby cheese and crema.

Serve with slices of avocado and tomato.

Fish Tacos

A homemade version of another favorite restaurant dish.

Make the sauce in a small bowl:

1 small Greek yogurt plain

¼ cup of mayonnaise

 chipotle sauce, add to taste, sauce will be pink in color

Squeeze of a fresh lime

Stir until blended.

Slice:

1/8 head of red cabbage into thin shreds.

Place on a plate:

2 corn tortillas

Some of the shredded red cabbage

In a skillet place:

2 Tablespoons olive oil

1 large or 2 small fish filets, any white fish

Cook until fish has turned white and opaque. It should flake with a fork.

Distribute the fish between the two corn tortillas and red cabbage. Top with sauce. Serve hot.

Serve with guacamole and baked chips.

Vegetarian Stir Fry

I made this on a day when I was too tired to defrost the shrimp. I grabbed a handful of walnuts out on the counter and threw them in. Now it is a favorite.

<u>Cut into bite sized pieces</u>:

1 Broccoli crown

2 Carrots, sliced thinly

4 oz. white mushrooms

1 16 oz. can of baby corn

Heat canola oil in a wok or deep sauté pan.

Place all the vegetables in the hot oil and cook until cooked but still firm.

<u>Add</u>:

½ bottle of stir fry sauce

Stir and allow to cook until well coated.

<u>Add</u>:

1 generous handful of raw walnuts

½ to 1 package of udon noodles

When noodles have softened, remove from heat.

Serve immediately. Makes enough for 2 people.

Pasta with Meat Sauce

A recipe my mom made when I was growing up. I changed it adding mushrooms and ground turkey.

Cook the pasta:

Bring to boil a 2-quart saucepan of water. When boiling, add 2 ounces of spaghetti pasta. Cook to desired softness. Place in a low soup bowl.

Make the sauce:

½ pound of lean ground beef or turkey

½ bell pepper

¼ small onion

2 cloves garlic, diced very small

4 ounces of white mushrooms, sliced

Cook the meat breaking it up as it cooks. Add the vegetables. Allow them to cook until just softened.

Add:

8 oz. of canned prepared tomato sauce

Allow to simmer.

Cook until all the vegetables are cooked soft and meat is cooked through.

Serve the meat sauce over the pasta noodles with freshly grated parmesan cheese and wheat garlic bolito bread slices.

French Bread Veggie Pizza

A homemade version of the frozen dinner packed with vegetables.

Cut a French bread loaf into thirds. Freeze two. With the remaining French bread slice it lengthwise and place on a foil lined baking sheet. Toast the bread in the oven.

<u>In a sauté pan, sauté together</u>:

¼ onion

½ bell pepper

4 oz. mushrooms

Cook until softened.

Place on the toasted bread:

Prepared tomato sauce to cover both halves of the bread

Sautéed vegetables

Tomato slices, sliced very thin

Freshly grated mozzarella cheese

Bake at 350 degrees until bread is crispy and cheese is melted.

Quesadillas

Another homemade version of a restaurant dish.

2 whole wheat tortillas

3 Chicken tenders, cooked and diced

Grated Colby cheese

Canned chilies

Brush a sauté pan with canola oil bring to heat. Place one tortilla in a sauté pan. Place on the tortilla the dice cooked chicken. Spoon on diced canned chilies to taste. Grate Colby cheese over the chicken and chilies, to just cover the chicken and chilies. Add another tortilla on top. Heat until cheese melts. Flip to cook the other side. It flips better if cheese touches both tortillas and melts together. Remove from the pan. Cut into wedges. Serve with tomato slices, avocado slices, and salsa.

Variation: you can substitute sautéed vegetables for the chicken. It is especially good with spinach.

Wraps

Got this from my daughter, who made them at work.

1 whole wheat tortilla

Hummus (I like the roasted bell pepper flavor)

Cucumber slices

Bell pepper slices

Baby spinach

Place the tortilla on a plate. Spread generously with hummus. Place cucumber slices in a row down the middle. Add bell pepper slices on the top, then the baby spinach. Roll up tightly. Cutting it in half makes it easier to eat.

Crock pot Chili

A favorite seasoning mix in Houston done my way.

False Alarm Seasoning mix

1 pound of ground lean beef or turkey

1 16 oz. can of unseasoned tomato sauce

1 16 oz. can of diced tomatoes

1 Cup of kidney beans, dried

Place all the ingredients in the crockpot except the salt and the masa. (I don't need the masa as a thickener because I don't add extra water.) Stir well mixing all the ingredients together. Cook on high in the crockpot for 4 hours.

Serve over ½ cup white rice and top with grated Colby cheese to garnish.

This will make several servings for company or to freeze and reheat later.

Sage Chicken Noodle Soup

I adapted this recipe from the work of Brother Victor-Antione d'Avila- Larourrette omitting the water and substituting sage for rosemary. I simplified it using only one kind of chicken and don't buy the pre-sliced vegetables. I added the crockpot method of dumping everything together at once. His recipe serves 10, this one 2.

<u>Place in a 2-quart saucepan or crock pot</u>:

½ small onion

1 stalk of celery, sliced

2 carrots, sliced thinly

Chicken tenders or skinless thighs, cut into bite sized pieces

32 oz. container of chicken broth

1 Tablespoon of dried sage

Cook on low until vegetables are done.

Add a handful of baby spinach

4 ounces of sliced mushrooms

A handful of dried pasta

Heat until vegetables are cooked and noodles are soft. About 7 minutes on the stove, 10 in the crock pot.

Serve with wheat bolito rolls and butter or margarine.

This makes more than one serving for sharing or saving.

Tikka Masala Meal (an Indian curry dish)

A homemade version of a favorite dish at an Indian restaurant on their buffet. Theirs is better. Chef Jamie Oliver recommended the brand of sauce.

Rice:

1 cup of water

½ cup of rice

Bring water to a boil. Add rice. Stir. Lower temperature to simmer. Place lid on. Allow to cook while preparing the rest of the meal.

Spinach side dish:

1 tablespoon canola oil

2 handfuls of fresh spinach

Cracked pepper

Garlic powder

Place canola oil and spinach in a sauté pan. Let cook down. Add pepper and garlic powder. Cook a little more. Place in 1/3 of a soup bowl.

Tikka Masala:

Tikka Masala curry sauce (Parak's)

Chicken tenders or thighs, cut into bite sized pieces

1 tablespoon Canola oil

In the same pan, place the canola oil and chicken pieces. Cook until browned. Add sauce, about half a jar. Stir. Lower heat and cover. Allow to simmer. When chicken is cooked through, add in the soup bowl. Add the rice.

Dressed Up Macaroni and Cheese

A friend of mine served me the Macaroni and cheese with broccoli in it when I went to her house. I added the tomatoes.

Make a box of macaroni and cheese. Use half the amount of butter or margarine and a little extra milk to make more sauce than the mix usually makes. Add 2 cups steamed broccoli and diced fresh tomatoes or halved cherry tomatoes. Stir. The extra sauce covers the vegetables.

Grown Up Grilled Cheese

A cheaper version of a sandwich I saw on the Oprah Winfrey Show. I added the tomato and avocado.

2 Sourdough bread slices

2 Provolone cheese

Butter or margarine

Tomato slices

Avocado slices

Honey

Dried basil

Butter the bread slices. Place one face down in a hot skillet. Place 2 slices of provolone cheese on the bread until the cheese gets soft. Remove from heat on to serving dish. Add tomato and avocado slices, a squeeze of honey and dried basil. Toast the other slice of bread in the hot skillet buttered side down. When toasted, place on top of the sandwich. Cut sandwich in half and serve.

Vegetable Plate

A restaurant in my area had a vegetable plate on their menu. I loved the idea and make them at home with my own vegetables.

Roasted vegetables have so much flavor. Cut up fresh ones that have approximately the same cooking time. You can determine this by noticing the density of the vegetables and group them and when you cut them up, cut them the same size. For ideas, notice what they mix together in the frozen section of the grocery store. Here are some ideas:

California mix: carrots, broccoli, cauliflower

Ratatouille: eggplant, onion, peppers, zucchini, tomatoes

You can roast individual vegetables too as a side. Whatever the case, toss them with healthy oil and herbs and spread them on a parchment lined baking sheet at 400 degrees.

Creamed vegetables taste good on a vegetable plate. Summer squash, winter squashes, or cauliflower cooked until very soft. Mash or put the vegetable through a ricer. Add a little milk, butter, salt and pepper.

Beans. Beans are a vegetable that add a protein to the vegetable plate. One popular type of bean here is the black eyed peas or the pinto beans.

Raw vegetables. Raw vegetables add crunch to the plate, something that adds variety of textures and color. Cold salads of different types like a tossed salad, a spinach salad, a cabbage slaw, and vegetable strips are all options of raw vegetables.

Be sure to include health fats, proteins, and fruits on the vegetable plate and you have a complete meal.

Shish Kebabs

We made this on the grill when I was a child.

Slide on to wooden skewers: Chunks of onion, fresh mushrooms, chunks of bell pepper, and chicken or beef cut in chunks. Sprinkle with salt and pepper. Add a BBQ sauce after grilling and meat is cooked, the last few minutes.

Taco Salad

We made this when I was a teenager. It was quite new at the time. I changed the recipe adding salsa to the meat, which was beef then, and adding avocado.

Ground turkey, cooked with salsa

Romaine lettuce, torn

Fresh tomato and avocado, diced

Grated Colby cheese

Individual bag of corn chips

Salad dressing, if desired.

Place ingredients in a bowl in this order: lettuce, cooked ground turkey, tomato and avocado, grated Colby cheese, corn chips. Add salad dressing if desired.

Portobello Mushroom Burgers

I had this at a hotel restaurant on a convention.

The Portobello mushroom replaces the hamburger in a regular hamburger type sandwich. You can grill the mushroom top whole or sliced. Place on a bun and top with fresh vegetables as you would a hamburger. Surprisingly filling.

◊◊◊

Recipes for Snacks

Baked Chips

I got this idea from a garnish for soup in a Richard Simmons recipe.

Cut 3 corn tortillas into 6ths. Place on baking sheet in a 350-degree oven. Let bake until crispy. Serve with guacamole or salsa.

Nachos

The school I worked at would make nachos this way for the children for snack sometimes. They used refried beans in their recipe. I added the guacamole and salsa.

Place baked chips in parchment paper lined baking sheet. Grate Colby cheese over the baked chips. Heat in the oven until melted. Top with guacamole or salsa.

Popcorn

Everybody made popcorn like this back in the day.

Make popcorn old-fashioned style on the stove. Kids will be amazed. I use a 2-quart saucepan that has a clear lid. Pour canola oil in the pan until it just barely covers the bottom of the pan. Sprinkle popcorn seeds to cover the oil in one layer. Place lid on. Heat over medium heat until the sound of the popping slows. Pour into a bowl. Add salt using a salt grinder. Serve immediately.

Cracker Snacks

More ideas from afternoon snacks at school.

Whole wheat crackers can be topped with peanut butter, sliced cheese, or cream cheese for a protein boost in the middle of the afternoon.

Jalapeno Poppers

A favorite of my daughter who convinced me to buy them prepared at the store to bake. My homemade version uses turkey bacon. Sometimes I don't blend the cheeses, just layer them.

2 fresh jalapeno peppers, large, split and seeded

Cream cheese

Grated Colby cheese

4 strips turkey bacon

Mix cream cheese and the grated Colby cheese. Spread cheese mixture into each half of the jalapeno peppers. Wrap each half with a strip of turkey bacon. Bake at 350 degrees until bacon is cooked and pepper is soft. Serve while warm.

Recipes for Desserts

A Taste of Cheesecake

Another afternoon snack idea from a school I worked at. They served graham crackers and cream cheese. My coworker suggested one day we at strawberries to make it taste more like pie. Everyone agreed.

Graham cracker

Spreadable cream cheese

Strawberry preserves

Spread graham cracker with cream cheese. Spread strawberry preserves over the top. It's a taste of cheesecake when I know I want the real thing.

Baked Fruit Crisps

My own version with less topping and more taste of the fruit.

Frozen mixed berries, one large apple OR one can of peaches in fruit juice

1 teaspoon of sugar if the fruit is too tart to your taste

Topping recipe: your favorite or purchased granola cereal

Oil a 4-inch diameter ramekin. Place fruit cut in bite sized pieces. Taste fruit. If it is too tart add sugar. If it is not, omit sugar. Sprinkle topping or granola on the top. Bake until bubbly. Let cool. Serve warm or cool.

Fresh fruit and Chocolate

Strawberries dipped in chocolate can be very pricey at the store. This has none of the preparation and all of the taste.

Your favorite fresh fruit

Chocolate: mini chocolate bars or kisses

On a plate, cut up fruit. Place a handful of chocolate. Eat slowly.

Fruit on Skewers

I had this for dessert in Boston after my first taste of lobster. I added the dip, a variation on a recipe I found in a cookbook. I don't blend anything into the yogurt.

Fresh fruit is fun to eat on wooden skewers and pretty with a variety of colors. Vanilla yogurt in individual bowls for dipping adds a flavor and texture contrast to the fruit that tastes good.

My Recipe Collection Notebooks

I have many more recipes I have cut out of magazines or scanned from cookbooks that I have or checked out of the library. I placed them in page protectors and organized them. I have four volumes: Everyday Recipes, Recipes to Try, Special Occasions & Sweets Stash, and My Family History Recipes. The two I use the most are the Everyday Recipes and the Recipes to try. These two notebooks contain lots of recipes featuring lean meats, fruits and vegetables and less breads and grains than I used to eat. The Special Occasions & Sweet Stash contain the recipes that are not for every day. These are the ones to impress guests or treat myself and the few sweets that I will make from time to time that I like the most. I used to eat a lot of sweets but not so much anymore. The family history recipes are from my past and they are the ones I do not use any more and organized according to the address of where I lived. The following paragraphs are specifically what is in these notebooks to help you in your search for new recipes of your own.

Everyday Recipes. There is a section on main courses with 24 recipes. These came from food magazines, women's magazines, books written by a catholic monk (they are known for being very frugal), the American Heart Association publications, mail order food kit recipes, and Weight Watchers publications.

I have 6 recipes that feature fish: a broiled fish recipe with a mayo and chive topping, a skillet dinner with vegetables, a broiled salmon with a honey mustard and dill topping, a sautéed salmon with tomato and capers, a baked fish with a light breadcrumb breading, and a fish baked in parchment with lemon and vegetables (green beans and mushrooms).

I have 6 meatless recipes: 2 with eggs and vegetables, 2 vegetable lasagnas, a vegetable stir fry, and a vegetable quesadilla recipe.

I have 4 pork recipes: one lightly breaded with breadcrumbs and sautéed, one in the crockpot with pineapple, one with a currant jelly sauce, and one sautéed with apples.

I have 3 shrimp recipes: one with couscous and vegetables, one with garlic and carrots, and one broiled with a variety of sauces.

I have 2 chicken recipes: one baked with cornflake crumbs and one with a Mexican green salsa.

I have one ground beef recipe: an adapted Japanese sukiyaki recipe.

Then there are the homemade versions of fast food and comfort food that is much healthier: turkey burger, sloppy joe, chicken nuggets, and red beans and rice. These use healthy oils, portion control, lower fat and sodium. They taste so much better when I want to eat fast food.

I have a section of 10 side dishes that are just vegetables both cooked and raw. Several roasted vegetables my favorite is the roasted ratatouille. A raw tomato and cheese salad with balsamic vinegar, a red cabbage slaw with apples and cranberries, a sautéed summer squash and lemon dish, broccoli salad, a fruit salad with honey and citrus, and a sautéed cauliflower and red pepper dish. There is also a chart on how to cook whole grains.

When I began this food journey I ate a lot of salads. Salads are the go to food for being healthy for many as well as me too. They are good hot weather food. I have 10 recipes including a crab salad in a cantaloupe half, spinach salad with orange dressing, a scallop salad with corn and avocado, chopped salads, tuna salad, and 5 dressing recipes.

Soups are a favorite too. They are nutrition in a bowl as I see it. I have 9 recipes: chicken noodle, shrimp gumbo, broccoli soup, ginger-carrot, onion, tortilla, beef stew, leek and potato, and Mexican corn. There are no cream soups. Some use skim milk.

I have a section of appetizers and desserts. I have 3 recipes: butternut squash wontons, crepes to put fruit inside, and fruit cup.

The last section is breakfasts: tortilla wraps, pancake recipes without white flour, pumpkin bread, wheat muffins, and an apricot oat bread.

The Recipes to Try notebook is not organized as the intention for those recipes is to try them and place them in the Everyday Recipes notebook. It contains 85 more recipes that are the same categories as the Everyday recipes. The ones I don't like will be discarded or passed on to someone else. There are some cool fruit desserts, soups, and more vegetables to try.

The Special Occasion recipes are for company and eaten only occasionally. I no longer eat from one holiday to another. In my collection is an egg and vegetable casserole for brunch, more recipes from the mail order food kits I want to simplify, 2 recipes for Bolognese tomato sauce, a vegetable tarte, lobster with wine sauce, sweet potato casserole, moo goo gai pan, tomato pasta, lemon garlic pasta, weeknight coq au vin, skillet baked spaghetti, and Pallela. These recipes are time consuming, have a lot of ingredients, or have expensive ingredients. I can't cook or eat like this every day. They are there to make someone feel special like for a birthday or other celebration.

I have 12 recipes in my <u>Sweet Stash</u>. This is way down from all I used to make. I kept my favorites: apple crisp and cookie recipes.

The holiday recipes I make only on the specific holiday. I sometimes choose from them and don't make all of them anymore. I don't eat them for the entire season anymore either. There are appetizers, food for New Year's Day, mint candy and fudge for Valentine's Day, Birthday cake recipes and frosting, and Christmas cookies and French Canadian Foods I make for Christmas Eve every year.

Things I Learned Along the Way

This is a collection of insights I had during the process. Take what you will from them.

Falling off the Wagon

Making mistakes are part of the process in learning anything. My biggest hurdle is comfort foods that remind me of good times and my favorites from childhood. I will add these in occasionally when I want them, and sometimes a little bit will do. Denying myself these foods only makes it worse. During holiday time, it is too easy to get way off and have to regroup and move forward back to healthy eating.

Sometimes, I found that I needed a recipe for a lighter version of these foods to satisfy. *Cooking Light* magazine is good about providing those recipes. Here are a few of mine:

Cheesy foods

Noodle and rice based dishes

Foods served with gravy or in gravy

Big pieces of meat

Rich desserts

Dips and chips

High fat picnic foods

I mentioned some of these in the wellness college class one time. One student said, "That's all the good stuff." I agreed. I also told them about the struggle of someone I knew had with trying to eat nine servings of fruits and vegetables a day and how hard it was to have to change it by doctor's orders, all at once. I got no response on that one.

It is better to plan a little taste of something I crave or even a meal of it and then get back to the healthy stuff than to white knuckle it until I am way off track. The longer I am off track the harder it is to get back as during the Christmas Holidays can be. Someone I know eats healthy all week then eats what he wants on the weekends. It works for him.

As I mentioned earlier, taking a little field trip to the healthiest places they serve or sell food might help, it does me. I have one place that makes smoothies out of fresh ingredients. When I want to get back on track, I go there. Just walking in the door the food smells so fresh that I want to start again. Same for the produce sections of a high end grocery. They too have processed foods so don't be fooled by that. Chips are chips no matter how much you pay for them. Fancy energy bars are usually more than one serving and can be more calorie dense than I need. Even fit people have to walk by these too.

Being too tired to cook is my best excuse. Sometimes I am just too tired. I try to keep a few simple meals at hand like sandwich ingredients or breakfast cereal for that. A 16-ounce cup of a fresh fruit smoothie with a protein boost can make me feel better in minutes. The store bought ones with a handful of raw nuts give me the same boost. Not having enough protein or vegetables gets me out of balance pretty quickly.

Being worried or stressed is my other excuse. Sometimes I put on a crock pot of food or get ingredients ready and go exercise. The stuff that bothers me gets burned off. When I come back, I am not as hungry and my home smells wonderful. Taking proactive steps to what is bothering me helps too.

Figuring out what the things are that causes me to fall off the wagon is sometimes no small task. Sometimes there are layers to pull back, finding something else to deal with under each one is in order. It is worth it to be healthier. I have done quite a bit of that. It proved to help a lot.

Making healthy choices can be super tough at times, it just can. Beginning again can make me feel good all over again. I have never become completely sedentary again since beginning. I have fewer and fewer blood sugar spikes where I get sleepy after eating. I feel so good I forget to test my blood sugar.

Processed Foods

Here is a list of the processed foods I ate from my menus notebook I don't use anymore. I put it together to help me remember what I served my kids and I. So often on shopping day I would draw a blank on what to get and serve. It was a resource notebook for me. This list is to give you an idea of what processed food is so that you can make better choices. Remember, the rule for healthy eating by Dr. Maya Adam is no processed foods at all.

Pocket type microwavable sandwiches

Calzones

TV dinners

Vienna sausages

Canned soups

Burritos

Bacon bits

Chicken patty

Egg sandwiches

Hot dogs

Dried noodle packets

Tater tots

Tamales

Lunch kits both refrigerated and non-refrigerated

Jar soups

Chips

Popcorn shrimp

Toaster pastries

French toast

Taco kits

Frozen waffles

Chicken pot pie

Taquitos

Deli meats

Travel soup cups

Frozen ravioli

Frozen lasagna

Turkey hot dogs

Canned pasta

Fish sticks

Corn dogs

Cheese in the shaker container

Cheese that does not need to be refrigerated

Dinner mixes

This list is not complete. If you disagree with anything on this list, please refer to the You Tube videos that explain the big business of food in the United States that Dr. Maya Adam explains so much better than I. Sometimes, the students in my classes were very unhappy to find this out and started arguments based on what they thought was good food. Food choices are a very personal issue. No one likes the feeling of someone taking something away they like. The trick of it is to replace the foods with homemade versions that you make yourself with fresh ingredients. It is not likely you will add preservatives, high fructose corn syrup, or hydrogenated oils to the foods you make yourself.

A Word About Stress

Stress is a big factor on the success of many things. It can be a motivator or a burden depending on how much of it there is. Stress influences blood sugar, it can make it worse.

There are these idealistic ideas in this culture I call "If only…". These are the ideas that if there was a major change like winning the lottery or retiring that they could be healthier and make it happen. Among these ideas are more money, more time, more motivation from family…the list goes on and on.

It fooled me too, no one of these things really do work. It took time to figure out what I wanted in my life. Money can't do that. Time can't do that. Other people cannot do it either. It has to come from within. It takes planning, willingness to make mistakes, and finding a balance for what I will and won't have in my life. It takes tenacity. It takes having to take responsibility for my own health. I know that if I had all this information while still working, I could have done better. I actually did use Dr. Adam's recipes while working and those worked out quite well.

I saw an older man looking around at recipe books in a bookstore for healthier eating when I was there the other day. He must have gotten overwhelmed. I saw him later in his pick-up truck, smoking. I see many people in the bookstore looking for the nutrition answer for themselves. Some ask the clerks who will help locate but not help decide. Some have family members they trust with them, the healthier one telling the other what to do. I have even been in a grocery store and seen fit looking health type professionals instructing people how to shop, with lots of talking and not much choosing. I have even been to a health food store and got cornered by an employee wanting to help me by selling me a lot of supplements who was sure if I bought his products I would most definitely be healthier (slimmer, actually). He made recommendations that did not consider the medications he didn't know I was taking and assumed I could afford to shop there. It was humiliating. I got a lot of stares in the healthier food stores too which is uncomfortable, at best. There are also doctors who use scare tactics. I am sure these things are true about what they say but knowing those things without the information and support made me feel powerless, not motivated. I just want to go home and make brownies after that, how about you? There are "friends" and family who intrude. I was overwhelmed. Then, when I lost the 56 pound, I became one of them so sure I had the answer. I didn't. I hated all of it and quit. I put all the weight back on. I didn't want to be like that. I wanted to be me, not an example. I didn't really know what to do.

Yet I know my quality of life has a steep price if I don't take care of myself. I run the risk of losing my legs or my eyesight to diabetes. With that comes mobility issues and the lack of freedom to pursue my own happiness, a really steep price. There are no guarantees. I have to be sure and live a life that I can take care of me. I personally had to make many changes to do that. I gave my whole life a makeover. I am very satisfied with what I have now. So is my doctor in regards to my health. I learned a lot. I am better. I got a stunned look the other day when I mentioned I could walk a 5K and did often. People like to assume they know the quality of my health by just looking at me. I know if I keep up with it, my body eventually will look better and possibly slimmer. The body responds to consistently good things. Less stress, more exercise, doing what I love, and good simple food is what is working for me.

It hasn't been an easy path in regards to the people in my life and the support I got. Some fought me to keep things the way they were in whatever means possible. I was undermined, tempted, and they brought in foods that are not good for a healthy life. I made changes slowly. I made it, served it, and adjusted it. They chose their favorites. I learned that making huge changes fast will make the problem bigger. We settled into some good habits and choices although not complete.

 Yes, there were people who did not change. One got instructions from a doctor to make the changes, years later. Others now make their own food choices and the responsibility is not mine anymore. Sometimes there is another issue that has nothing to do with getting healthy that is involved. I decided to relieve my own pressure valve.

I have discovered that stress is sometimes like junk mail. You just have to go through it regularly and toss it out. This world dishes it out in portions under many disguises. I personally had to be brave and go for it.

My First 5K and Exercise Tips

It was a 5K that happened at night with glow powder and black light stations. I decided I wanted to go when I learned they accepted people who walked. It had a before party with loud music to get everyone excited when I got there. It worked. It was exciting. After a while, I got thirsty for water and there was no free water. In August. In Houston. Go figure. I had to walk back to my car to get money. (I ended up walking two 5Ks that day because my car was parked so far away.) I thought that I was going to be the last one to finish the race when I went, that everyone was going to be fit but me. I decided to do it anyway. I knew I could do it, I walked one every day. I decided it was okay to finish last.

What I found was people who did not walk at all. One woman, at least 400 pounds sitting was with her family in the heat, sweating. I was so afraid for her. I said a prayer for her about not walking today at this event she was clearly not ready for. I found more people that sat and smoked. How would they do it? I wondered. Then there were the lean ones who clearly this event was too easy for them, as I expected. And everyone in between including children in strollers with their families.

I ended up about 50 feet from the starting line. A woman who was in front of me with her adult daughter went down from the heat, not passing out, but clearly in some kind of distress. She was revived with the help of medics and water. It was August in Houston, at sunset, the hottest time if the day, the hottest time of the year, on concrete. A hush went over my part of the line.

Everyone checking themselves and loved ones. Then we were off.

The fit ones ran the course. I knew I was going to get passed up by a lot of people. I figured it was about 85% of them when it was all over. It was a little disheartening. The music they used to pump us up earlier was playing. I was in my normal pace. Smokers were breathless and smoking on the sidelines. I stopped for water and a wanted a picture of myself at a black light station. I traded my phone with a man who took my picture and I, his trading our own phones.

"This is really far," he said.

"I walk a 5K every day," I replied.

"You do?"

"Yes, sometimes all at once and sometimes half in the morning and half at night."

"Oh," he replied. Just as I suspected, some of the people here thought they could walk a 5K without training for it.

"It is on my bucket list." I replied. Now he was intrigued. He walked with me quite a long way trying to squeeze out of me what else was on the bucket list and complaining the course was too long. I didn't tell him what was on my bucket list. When he discovered I did not want to date him, I walked the rest of the course alone.

I finished the course. No one was at the finish line for me. It felt really good just the same. I took a picture and had others take a picture of me with glow powder on me and my number proudly on my t-shirt. Even today if I hear the song "Summer" by Calvin Harris, it all comes back at what I accomplished. I still walk nearly every day, though I listen to my body and walk less when I am tired and walk a 5K 3 or 4 times a week.

Exercise Tips:

Here are a few things I discovered about exercising after not doing so for a long time:

I plan to exercise near bathrooms. I discovered everything gets "moving" and it will be more frequent regardless of what I do for exercise. The weightlessness in the water can trick me into thinking I have a little longer than I do.

I take it at my pace not what someone else says. I am not making a tv show. I am making a life. The longer it takes to put it in place, the longer it sticks.

I am not into the notion of "no pain, no gain". Hurting myself only puts me back on the couch. I don't want to do that. Soreness bothers me afterwards, sometimes. At first I took medication for pain, then I decided to try water like a hot shower or hot tub. It is enough most days. In winter, I found water to be too drying on my skin, so I tried an electric blanket. Very cozy.

I learned how to lace my shoes to prevent squeaking and slipping. I was getting blisters and discovered the directions in websites for runners. Cleared up my foot problems.

Injury is part of overdoing it. It can set me back. I felt a surge of energy one day and decided to go with it. I walked seven miles in a day both days in one weekend. It felt so good. When I went out on the Monday following, I got a new sensation in my left foot. My toenail fell off. I went to a doctor at an emergency clinic and he said, "What did you do that for?" He told me to take it easy for a couple of days and go see a specialist. The specialist trimmed away most of my toenail. I told him about the pain on my heel while too. I ended up in orthotics and a night brace with medication for pain. I asked him if I could go back to walking. He said to take it easy. I went out and made it halfway around the block. Lucky for me there was a shortcut there. I came home and cried. I would have to start all over again, slowly. My plans to be in my first 5K in March were over. I healed and went slowly, my first 5K was in August. I take it easier these days. That toenail still tingles when I am doing too much. I always stop when that happens so I don't lose it again. Good news for me is that it is healed and I am in heels again by the company of shoes my doctor recommended. Going slowly matters.

Trip to the Healthiest City

I went to a convention for work. Something was really different about this city I was visiting. I noticed it right away. There were lots of fit people everywhere. I looked up my hunch on the internet. I was spending four days in the healthiest city in America. I was from the city that got to be the country's unhealthiest cities three years in a row. What an eye opening experience it was.

I ate twelve meals there but it was much more than the food offerings. There was a whole different way of living that I struggled with at home that didn't happen here. They purposely made it healthy and didn't offer anything else. The lack of temptation made healthy living easier. I wanted to take it home with me.

Specifically, there were bicycles everywhere. If you didn't have one, you could rent one for the day and leave it off at one of the many stations around the city when you were finished. There were bicycle paths everywhere and people seemed to ride very safely. In my city, we have bicycle paths too but it is not bicycle friendly. It is every man for himself in the traffic with a car, let alone on a bicycle. We have a once a month bike ride in downtown on a Sunday where they shut down some streets. The camp is divided between those that want to go ride and those that are annoyed by the closed streets. They have since installed many bicycle stations like the ones in the city I visited, where I live but it is not wide spread. There is a growing number of bike paths but not all are safe.

In that city the public transportation is all electric busses. There are no diesel fumes there to breathe like in my city.

In that city there are lots of places to walk, some of them very protected from the weather. The excuse in my city is that we have terrible weather. Theirs is equally as terrible and they make provision for it.

In regards to the food where I was, there were no fast food restaurants near where I stayed. Fruits were served in servings as much as three times the size I can get at home in restaurants. Vegetables were offered at every meal. I was only offered French fries once. I said no thank you. He offered me other choices of fruits and vegetables. I went to a shop that served sandwiches and coffee and smoothies. I took a sandwich out of the cooler and took it to the counter. The lady said, "You have a sandwich." I expected her to say, "Would you like chips and a drink?" (Where I live "drink" is code for soda pop.) The pause made me look for the chips. There were none in sight and no soda either. I chose a smoothie. Later, I looked at this little place closer and I did see chips, they were up high and in a corner on a shelf. I did notice that they offered bottled water, tea, and sports drinks. This was pretty much the norm everywhere. There was no candy out everywhere. The only candy I saw for sale were these little chocolates that looked like little pieces of art. You could buy them by the piece. They were too pretty to eat. Off in the corner on the side in the back was the candy I was familiar with. I noticed too that there weren't any doughnuts offered at the coffee shop. There were lot of muffins and quick bread slices. There were lots of choices of things with no frosting on them.

I did splurge there and order dessert, chocolate cake. I didn't know what I would get. He brought out a lovely little plate of 2, ½ inch slices of cake about 2 X 3 inches with a squeeze of chocolate sauce and a few raspberries. It also had a small dollop of whipped cream about 2 tablespoons. I was so surprised; it took my breath away. The server asked me if it was okay. I told him it was wonderful and proceeded to tell him about the size of cake in restaurants in my city. I told him about the slices they sell that are as much as 6 inches tall and 4-inch-wide wedges that they make it seem okay by giving two forks for sharing. He couldn't believe it. This restaurant could serve four people with what I could get at a restaurant at home.

I got to thinking about all of this when I got home. What a difference it would make if there were no French Fries, soda, chips or candy readily available in my city. What if it were not an option? What if we took away the excuses and temptations and made it possible and easier to be healthy like this city? I walked into my grocery store when I got home and there were mounds of sweets with lots of frosting right as you walk inside the door. I went to a restaurant and I was one of the average sized people in there, back at home. Many were much larger than me. Could it be that we are accustomed to this and it is normal for us? There has to be a new normal. The problem is much more complex than all of this but this is a good place to start.

I am not one to blame government. I consider myself an agent of change. If I don't buy it, they may stop offering it when others stop too. Business is relatively simple. They offer what sells. In some places there are government interventions. Good for them. I am not waiting on that. I also now have a great place to vacation in the summer, if I so desire.

It was uncomfortable to be one of the biggest people there. There was only one other than me who made sushi but it was welcoming there just the same. They are very patient with the people that attend conventions there. They teach by example.

Eating Out at Restaurants

Eventually better days will come when my income will permit me to spend more on food. I am working towards that now. I have decided to make a plan for that, when it comes.

It will be very easy to eat out again, an option that can be a minefield of nutrition mistakes for me. Some restaurants are for a treat. Some are for every day. Some indulge guilty pleasures. Some claim to do everything well. Some have signature house dishes. Portion sizes vary from teeny tiny to feeding a family of four. What to do?

Here are a few of my favorite healthy restaurant foods:

Salad bars: have a variety of fresh fruit and vegetable choices. They can't hide that it wilts or changes in the air on the table. You can regulate how much dressing you put on it. They offer soups and baked potatoes where I live on salad bars too.

Soup: most soup is cooked somewhere else and shipped to the restaurant chain in plastic bags. I try to order a clear broth soup. Homemade soup is available anytime because they make a big pot of it that has been simmering for hours. The vegetables still have some firmness to them and in generous amounts.

Sandwich: these are a quick meal out. The best places make it fresh just for me, using lean not deli meats, and fresh vegetables on whole grain breads or mixed flour breads.

Homemade food: not from a chain restaurant unless it is obvious they made it or let you assemble it or let you see them prepare it.

Pho: A big bowl of Asian noodles. The clear broth is very tasty and you can add fresh ingredients that they serve with it.

Dumplings: steamed dumplings in a bamboo basket steamer with lots of sauces is a great food adventure if you get the mixed order of fillings. It can come with soup. Lots of fun.

Half portions: some restaurants are glad for to let me order a half portion to split with a friend. They will even make both plates look good.

Buffets: These can be another minefield or a blessing depending on how I choose. It is way cheaper than ordering a la carte when I can choose the freshest vegetables, fruits and lean meats.

Healthy items marked on the menu: many restaurants have special items marked on the menu and how many calories it is. Sometimes they feed me nicely. Sometimes they starve me with this.

A meal of appetizers: I was at a restaurant that had healthy appetizers so me and the person I was with shared 3 orders. It was fun to taste everything.

Eat at home, go out for dessert: I can eat lighter at home and go for a treat like ice cream. It's fun with walking afterwards.

My plan for home food preparation for better days when I have a higher income is this: I will stop shopping at the dollar store and buy higher quality produce and lean meats, maybe even that ahi tuna. I would like to try those boxed meal kits of fresh ingredients that come shipped to my door. I have tried them at someone's house before. It tastes like healthy restaurant food. The ingredients come whole and fresh as they promise. It is an option for when life gets busy again. I will continue to follow this plan I made for me and monitoring my blood sugar. I have come too far to pretend I don't know.

Kid Food Craze

While I was eating lunch with my eleven-month-old grandson, I remembered during my own children's upbringing the heavy marketing to children that was going on to children through children's TV. It cost me more to buy these special foods. They loved the packaging and the hype. When I took them to the grocery store, these items were at child eye level. They had to have these items loaded with sugar and colorings. The packaging had cartoon characters on them.

They didn't always eat these foods. When they were very young, I gave them fruit, vegetables, granola bars, yogurt, lean meats, breads among some processed foods. The kindergarten teacher said I packed some very healthy lunches for my kids. They ate them until they saw what others were eating. That is when the kid food craze hit the hardest.

In my upbringing, we had a family dinner in which everyone was present and ate the same thing. I decided to revisit that with my kids. I left them home during this kid food craze at my house and did my food shopping alone unannounced. It went from disappointment of not getting these foods to be coming a "magic" refrigerator that food just appeared in. I knew I had achieved the right mindset in them when one of them opened the refrigerator and said, "We have food!"

Today, my grandson is starting table food and I am confident to offer him the foods I eat that are in this book. His eyes light up when he sees the brightly colored foods like strawberries on vanilla yogurt in a parfait glass. He is very interested in what his mom and I are eating and willing to taste it. He has had the sage chicken soup put through a food processor, turkey burger, and the baked sweet potato fries. I am delighted that his mom chooses healthy foods for him and herself. I am glad we have rejected the kid food craze. Children's television is cooking with vegetables and fruits these days instead of candy, chips, and sweets.

Both my children as adults have returned to their earlier food habits as I had hoped. I knew the early years in a child's life set up powerful patterns that I had learned in my work in early childhood education and stays with them. I am pleased. They both cook for themselves and share photos of food they have prepared with each other.

So the kid food craze didn't last. My grandson now has a great beginning too.

Onward

At this point, this goal of healthy eating and living might be overwhelming to you, my reader. It was for me too. As I build it, it eventually became routine. I had to quit and start many times before I was satisfied with the results. Many things are like this in life. Know that my quality of life is up to me and yours up to you. I wish you much success as you puzzle out what works for you.

Be good to yourself in the process of taking good care. Taking a gentle approach with yourself that didn't know, is better than an internal war. We all live and learn and different times and different ways. I hope this has been helpful to you.

Hope to see you out on the path, the walking path, that is.

Susan

◊◊◊

Additional Sources

Just in case you want to know a little more about some topics I mentioned in the book.

The **textbook** I used when I taught the course "Wellness of the Young Child" at the community college: Robertson, C. (2010) Safety, Nutrition, and Health in Early Education. Thomson Delmar Learning: Clifton Park, New York. 4th Edition. It is for child care providers and has more than nutrition information.

A list of companies started during the Great Depression: http://www.mtclaw.com/businesses_started_during_depressio n.html

More about **Coursera**, the platform of free courses: coursera.org. These are college level courses that would be the equivalent of an online continuing education course and many colleges and universities. Not all the courses are offered all the time.

My **favorite Dr. Maya Adam videos**: They are on YouTube. Child Nutrition and cooking 47 course videos on a playlist. Just click and settle in. It is a short version of the course I took. There is another part of her channel titled: Stanford Introduction to Food and Health with more technical information, if you so desire, with lectures of diagrams she draws as she speaks. The lecture I was referring to as big business in my introduction is actually titled "Industrial Agriculture", a must-see. If you get in the course and on the e-mailing list, she will direct you to all the other things she has going on.

More about **measuring food servings with your hand**: http://www.colormehealthy.com/0_docs/ServingSizeInHand.pd f. This is a diagram that explains this simple idea.

More about locating **5K races** near you: Active.com has lists of races to participate in. They are not free. You do get a shirt and number and bragging rights for the fee if you sign up early.

More about **shoes with support** for everyday: Crocs.com. Unbelievable, huh. They got together with podiatrists to design the best shoes for your feet. They have more than the ugly clog. I found some cute ones and some flip flops that are doctor approved. Not all their designs have support. Try them on. You will see what I mean.

More about **mail order food kits**: Blue Apron, Hello Fresh, and so many more. Once you click on one, you get the ads for the others.

About the Author

Susan Devine Napoli is a retired early childhood education professor and teacher of young children. Keeping children is healthy is always a concern of parents and caregivers alike. In teaching the class Wellness of the Young Children, it gave her insight and a desire continue with her search for healthy eating and living when she was not working.

She also spends time at her studio in a public office building where she does her creative work including writing, painting, and altered couture. She enjoys tiny living with her cat Dani. Who would rather sleep on a heating pad or eat.

She is online at: **SN Books Facebook page** and has a new **website on Google sites titled SN Books and Art**. It is there you can see all her creative projects and how to buy them.

Susan has been writing since 1980.

www.ingramcontent.com/pod-product-compliance
Lightning Source LLC
Chambersburg PA
CBHW071216280526
45787CB00002B/701